I0488198

Eyes of the Fat Man

Eyes of the Fat Man

How to Lose Weight for Good
No more phony diets

Randy Martin, MD

Writers Club Press
New York Lincoln Shanghai

Eyes of the Fat Man
How to Lose Weight for Good

All Rights Reserved © 2003 by Randy Capocasale

No part of this book may be reproduced or transmitted in any form or by any means, graphic, electronic, or mechanical, including photocopying, recording, taping, or by any information storage retrieval system, without the written permission of the publisher.

Writers Club Press
an imprint of iUniverse, Inc.

For information address:
iUniverse
2021 Pine Lake Road, Suite 100
Lincoln, NE 68512
www.iuniverse.com

No part of this document may be transmitted, stored in a retrieval system, or reproduced electronically or mechanically, including, but not limited to photocopies, photographs, slide, overheads, and magnetic tapes and disks, without prior written permission from the publisher.

ISBN: 0-595-26912-5

Printed in the United States of America

PREFACE

EYES OF THE FAT MAN is about the surgical procedure called gastric bypass or gastric reduction or gastrostomy or gastric resection or stomach stapling. My story is hope. It is for people who need to lose weight and thought it impossible. The procedure is not inaccessible, impractical, or beyond your reach.

People don't need another diet book (that's exploitation). They do need to know about gastric reduction. They need first hand information. Unfortunately, their doctors aren't telling them.

I should have known about gastric reduction ten years ago. I thought it was only for the most extreme cases, and that it was difficult to manage. I was just plain uninformed. There are millions of people like me as the emotional and physical disorder of obesity is endemic. Maybe I can wake you up.

Randy Martin, MD
9 October 99

CONTENTS

CHAPTER 1—LEARNING TO BE FAT

I learned I was fat when I was four. Fairmont School stood like a monument at the end of our street, Mayfair Boulevard. Some of us that afternoon, had gone over to play. In front of the main office, with its huge glass plate, was a little concrete bunker. We jumped in pretending it was our fox hole. Today we'd tired of that and made a pile of leaves, brown and dry. It was fall and we had moved in July, arriving in Columbus on the first, my birthday. It was all new to me. I had spent the first four years of my life in apartments in Padua and Bologna. I was still an only child. My brother would be born next year and these were my first playmates. A few new kids arrived. Some little girl said, "You're fat." A little chorus chimed in, "He's fat." and then with, "Randy's fat, Randy's fat."

The sting was unbelievable, and had the suddenness of death. The rejection and condemnation rang in their voices. What had I done? They told me I was bad, and they barely knew me—not like my parents, and especially my mommy. If that horrible thing were true, they would have told me. They loved me and would have told me and protected me and corrected it, especially if it were such a horrible thing.

My pain turned to rage, and I fired back. "I'm not fat! I'm medium!" and blind with anger, I could find nothing to throw at them but dry leaves—an impotent gesture.

I went home and told my mother, saying, "They said I was fat. I'm not, I'm medium, aren't I?" which I truly believed. I think she agreed, and I asked her, "Mom, could I have some scrambled eggs?" Dad was away that night, at his residency, and we would not eat together that evening.

The hurt of that event was repeated many times in childhood, and it always stung just as much. And each time, it knocked my love for myself further down. I could never fully be the good guy or somebody's hero. Being an object of laughter and ridicule however, I developed humor as a tool, that is, directed the laughter toward myself (It was gratifying to be able to make people laugh.) and at the same time, directed the ridicule elsewhere, away from myself. There was some malleability then in people's reaction to me and my shame. And it was a good intellectual exercise always to try to be funny. The first time I remember purposely doing so in school was when I squatted like an ape bouncing up and down, and scratching under my arms. It drew good laughs in the coat room, out of sight of Miss Miller. Then there was the gag on TV: the advertising jingle said, "Winston tastes good, like a cigarette should." And a young woman chewed and swallowed her cigarette. I imitated that for Miss Miller with a rolled up piece of paper, and got a luke warm response. The act of performing became itself compensatory, and in front of the Lazarus Santa Clause I was irrepressible, singing and dancing.

It always stung just as much. My best friends were Richard and Robert Hershberg, whom I'd met the first year in school. Before I knew them, my mother and I were taking one of our long walks back from the stores on Broad Street. One of the play grounds caught my eye because of its large beautiful bank of swings and its extra tall slide. I asked my mom if I could play with them, she said yes, and as I approached, they said, "Here comes fat old Randy." I thought I would turn around, but I said no, I must go on. I said to myself, "I want so badly to be friends with them, and anyone else would tease me worse. I have to make friends sometime, even if I must swallow such a big piece of my pride." And I played with them and they seemed sorry for having called me that and they were kinder, and more pitying than the other children. The Hershbergs—they were Jews who had escaped from communist Hungary, and they were a lovely family. They had a sister, Sharon, who was fat, fifteen, and sweet as could be, and an older brother, Eric, who was tall, thin, and athletic. He would play with us, setting up little Olympic games and teaching us everything and anything he'd learned. And I thought he knew everything, and was flattered. Richard was a year older than Robert. They looked alike, had brown curly hair, wore glasses and had goofy affable smiles. We became steadfast friends, to my heartache, when we left, on my birthday, when I was eight. I remember Sharon asking me, "Aren't you sad to be leaving us?" My seven year old brain answered, "I didn't cry when my grandmother died." since that was the saddest thing I had seen happen in my young life. (I remember being amazed and dismayed that I couldn't feel what the adults were feeling; and so I gave her that specimen of my toughness almost as a question.) She said, "Well you should cry now." I wouldn't then, but I'm crying at the thought of it now

We moved to Zanesville, and here the challenge of again gaining friends and fighting the isolation of obesity started all over. And it marked nearly every relationship with ambivalence and distrust. Sooner or later I might be teased by a friend which stung even more since it carried the venom of betrayal: Sooner or later when the social climate would change and the spirit of mob or committee prevail. All my trust lay in a few loving and trustworthy individuals and never in society at large. Even Margie and David Johnson who lived across the alley from us and whom I had befriended one summer night by giving them a firefly I'd caught, started in on me one evening and that mean crew cut bastard from across the street who was three years older presented himself and denounced me as fat. The metaphors, similes, analogies and hyperbolizes persisted so long and I refused to give ground so long that my father had to come out and say, "Why do you disturb him, he doesn't eat your food." And Margie Johnson being the pretty little blond girl who played the piano and was well behaved told me in a goody two shoes way that I instantaneously despised that my father was right, I didn't eat her food and said she was sorry for teasing me.

And in school, life went on with the usual remarks, such as the one from Monty Perry, "You don't mind if we call you Tubby, do you?" to which I politically said no, while my blood boiled. I minded very, very much, and he knew it. But there wasn't a thing I could do…

Save diet. I started dieting at an early age—eight. Actually, I thought of it when I was seven, but the idea of quantity wasn't part of it. My original idea was that certain foods made you fat. For example, my father had told me that sweets and candy would make you fat, and he had pointed out a fat boy eating a chocolate bar saying, "See, he eats the wrong foods." And so I remember one morning when I was seven, and having breakfast, and my father called, and I asked him, "Dad, will farina (cream of wheat) make you fat?" He said no. Did he add, "…unless you eat too much?" I can't recall.

Around eight, the idea of quantity entered into it: I remember deliberately eating less at dinner and then being hungry at night, and repeatedly pilfering quartered slices of American cheese on squares of soda crackers. Nothing I did changed my chunky physique…

Until gym class at Roosevelt Junior High. Between the ages of twelve and fourteen, I gradually, miraculously thinned, and at fifteen, I was six foot and 165 pounds—just about right, though my fellows never let me forget I was actually fat. I stayed thin until my last two years of college when I buckled down in New York City. Sedentary and studious, I gradually rose to 210. I was shocked and saddened and over the next three years literally starved myself down to 156 pounds by age twenty-five. I considered it a splendid effort, but really no match for the strains of marriage and applying to medical school. I gained it all back and a little more. My weight of 215 led to many an embarrassing interview before admissions committees—hardly professional, and no doubt cost me slots. In the misery of medical school, I gradually worked my way up to an astounding 245 by means of hospital cafeterias and late night vending machines. Just as I finished school, I had a near fatal head on collision in the desert of Umatilla, Oregon. I had fractured my feet and my left leg was in a Hoffman device. By the time I could start my residency, six months later I was up to 270 or so. Extraordinary! I never thought it could happen to me, and very embarrassing. In my first years of practice in the sedentary specialty of psychiatry I gradually achieved 300 pounds—my true low point—and food was good wherever I went. I would diet, lose 10 pounds and gain it back and would never get my swimming in. Finally I tried a modified fast , a nightmarish ordeal, and got back to 270 pounds. Then three years ago, developed my first diabetic symptoms and about a year later lost around 10 pounds from diabetes. Then I heard a surgeon talk about gastric reduction....

Chapter 2—THE PROCEDURE

Armstrong wants to specialize in this operation when his stint in the Army's done. The presentation he gave to the medical staff went like this:

Statistically, medicine's attempts at weight reduction in the truly obese have been dismal. People may succeed in losing 20 to 30 pounds and in keeping it off. 40 to 60 pounds is much more questionable and at eighty and above, it is definite that the weight is likely to stay, despite repeated loss. Actually above 20 pounds, if weight is lost, it's likely to be gained back; and in someone who remains serious about dieting, there is likely to be a cycle of weight gain and weight loss. Below 30 pounds, that is of much less physiological detriment. In fact, it has been shown on reappraisal of Metropolitan Life's weight norms that people who were some 10 percent overweight lived the longest. So it may be a healthy tendency to gain that extra 10 percent which translates to 15 to 20 pounds or it may simply be a concomitant factor. That is, people who gain that little extra weight may have other advantages in life.

But the discouraging fact, demonstrated repeatedly in diverse statistics is that weight lost (particularly over 30 pounds) will be gained again. At excess weights of 30 pounds or under, that is of little impact. At greater excess weights it's much greater. It means that dieting alone is of proven limited significance. The so-called "change of lifestyle" is just further extension of dieting. Essentially all combined behavioral methods—change in exercise, activity and intake are ineffective in any meaningful way in dealing with excesses of 30 pounds. Surely there are exceptions but rare.

These are just the statistics. What's left? Diet pills. These are all amphetamines of one kind or another. They're all addictive—drawback enough. What do the stats show? The following: that people lose on average 20 pounds while taking amphetamines and gain 20 pounds back when they stop taking them. You could keep taking them and then run into the problems encountered using addictive stimulants. Basically, addictive substances are harmful to the central nervous system. Amphetamines in particular run the metabolism at high speed. Used chronically they produce an attention deficit syndrome and the person who has used them for years often appears jittery, distracted and has difficulty focusing. Stimulants like amphetamines and cocaine cause muscle to spasm. The small arteriolesat a the distal end of the circulation are lined with muscle. Arterioles supplying brain tissue when exposed to stimulantsn spasm and when they do so cause very small strokes because blood trapped at the spasming site clots just as blood shaken in a test tube will clot. It is the same mechanism that accounts for heart attacks in well trained atheletes who used cocaine before their death. The brain of a heavy user of stimulants or cocaine when viewed on MRI shows many pinpoint spots of light—the sites of these microstrokes—that give it the so called moth eaten appearance.

A maladaptive pattern of substance use, leading to clinically significant impairment or distress, as manifested by three or more of the following occurring at any time in the same twelve month period.

For a minority of amphetamine users dependency will also be a problem. As is well known dependency means tolerance and or withdrawal symptoms. Tolerance is the need for more and more of the substance to achieve the same gratification. Withdrawal is the body's physiological response to sudden absence of the substance. In the case of alcohol or benzodiazepines these may be delusions, hallucinations, even seizures. Withdrawal symptoms are often thought of as the opposite of the effects of the substance so that people withdrawing from amphetamines may feel slowed down and sleepy, may have difficulty concentrating and may have an increase in appetite. People who are dependent may often not only continue using for the primary gratification of the substance but also from sheer fear and avoidance of withdrawal. Other symptoms of dependency are the utter powerlessness to resist using, using more than intended, giving up important activities or opportunities, spending too much time obtaining or using the substance, and finally the added shame of that powerlessness in that the person is aware of his self destruction—of the bodily, social, occupational harm the substance does—but continues to use, in fact has usually failed repeatedly at heroic efforts to stop.

That is, for 20 pounds of weight loss the cure can be worse than the disease.

These facts should affect those people hawking diets or peddling diet pills—a large financial interest. That includes a range from those working off of their kitchen table selling homemade remedies by mail order to billion dollar drug companies sprawled out on acres with buses to carry staff from complex to complex. Unless of course, they somehow come up with a pharmacological miracle. But how could they? If satiety depends on filling the stomach, and if the stomach is instinctively geared to be stuffed, and the availability of food is limitless? What drug, or what paten table device, will convince the stomach it's full when it isn't; or convince the brain the stomach's full when it isn't? Someday it may happen.

For now, what's left? Gastric reduction—surgically reducing the size of the stomach. Statistically, people undergoing this procedure lose seventy pounds (on average) and as a rule, those pounds stay off.

The first bypass operations were at the University of Iowa in 1966. The stomach was transected into a small upper segment and a large lower segment. Part of the small intestine was then hooked to the upper segment to form a new pathway. The bypassed lower segment continued to function normally, but did not receive food.

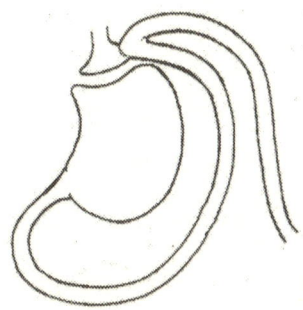

One variation of that procedure has been to staple rather than transect the stomach, and make the same join with the small intestine and upper segment.

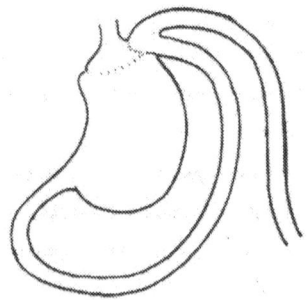

Another gastric reduction has been the vertical banded gastroplasty. Nearly all the stomach is stapled "out of the loop," stapling it almost closed. It is simple, safe, and doesn't disturb the rest of the digestive pathway, but for many patients, there is inadequate weight loss and persistent reflux.

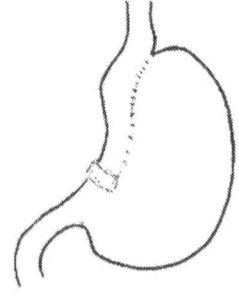

Currently two versions of transection or trans-stapling are common: the proximal and the distal Roux-Y gastric bypasses.

The proximal Roux-Y places a length of intestine between the small gastric pouch and the rest of the intestines that is less than forty inches, and connects to the intestine just below the stomach—that is, within eight inches, leaving about 15-16 feet of intestine available for absorption.

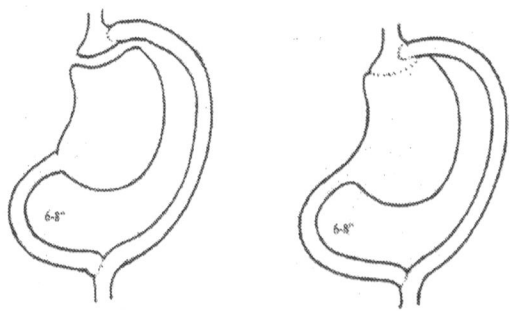

It works solely by encouraging effective dieting. That is the upper pouch holds 2-3 tablespoons of food, and further, the new opening between upper pouch and small intestine is narrow, about 1/2" in diameter. That slows the passage of food and further adds to rapid and sustained satiety

The distal Roux-Y is much more than an aid to dieting as not only the stomach, but also most of the small intestine is bypassed. The segment connecting the small gastric pouch to the remainder of the intestine is about sixty inches. The segment of intestine from the large gastric pouch is about six to eight feet. That leaves about forty inches of intestine available for absorption.

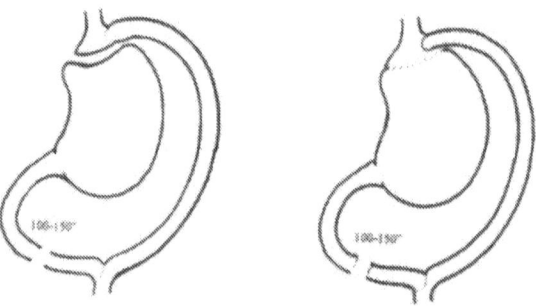

It leads to more weight loss than proximal bypass, but to more abdominal cramps, flatulence, diarrhea, protein and vitamin malnutrition, osteoporosis and ulceration, all of which, by the way, can be avoided by taking the proper precautions.

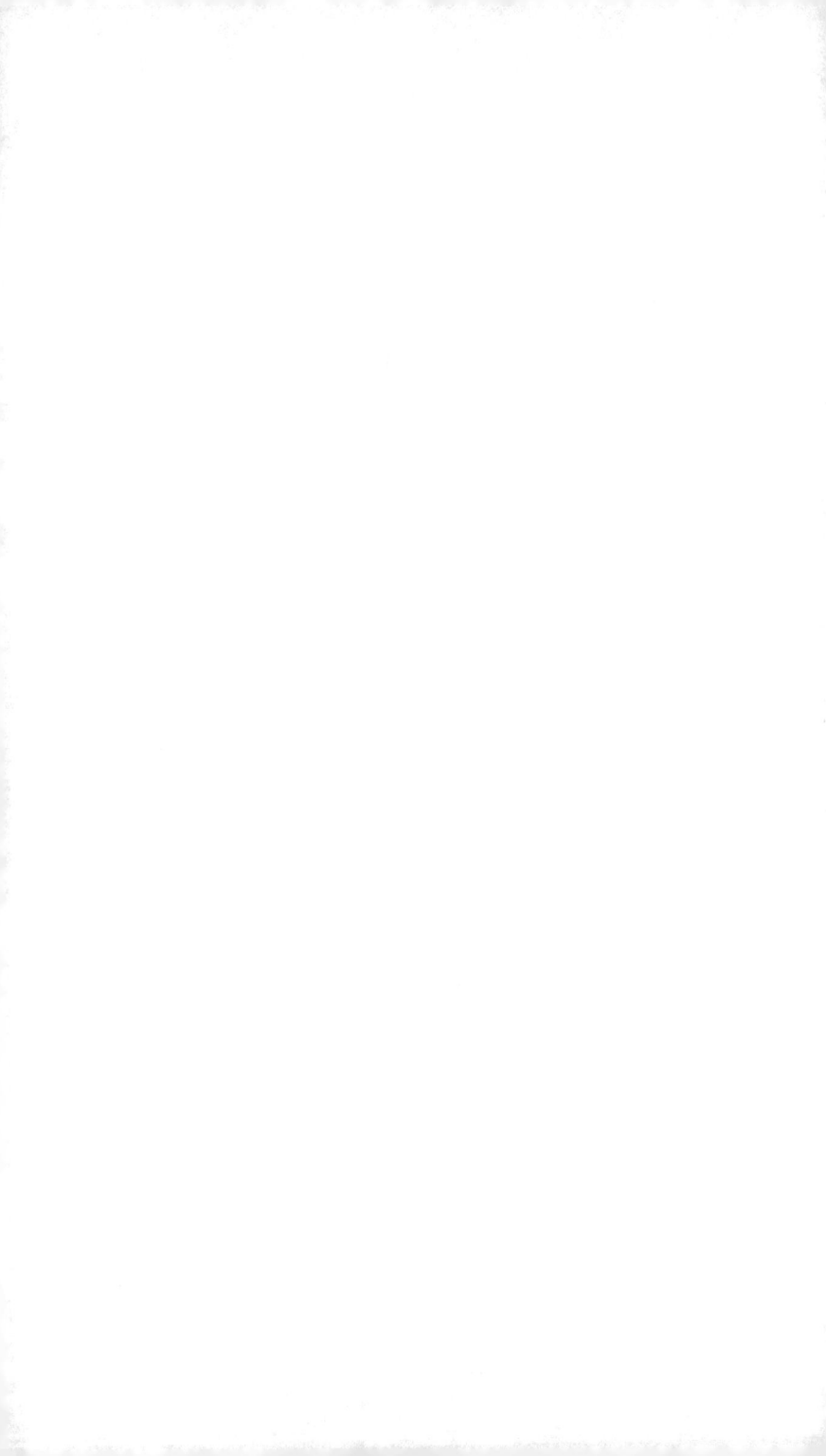

Chapter 3—DEPENDENCE OR OBESITY

The soldier sat down. He was about twenty.

"How are you?"

"Fine"

"How long have you been doing the program?"

"Two months."

"How long have you been abstinent?"

"Ten days."

"Good. (Pause) What's your understanding of alcohol dependency?"

"…It means…you can't live without drinking."

Or "It means you have to drink to feel normal."

Or "If you don't drink, you get sick."

"Good. But it's a medical condition. It's not just a behavior. It's as real as a broken leg."

Perplexed looks. (What does this guy want?)

"Alcohol dependency is an inherited neurological condition that declares itself in your early twenties. Biologically, that's all it is. It's not what people think; it's not a moral weakness, or some kind of corruption, or laziness, or degeneracy, or lack of will power. People are eager to criticize. Don't let them put you down. It is inherited, that is, nearly always there is at least one first degree relative with the condition. What precisely is inherited? It is the excessive release of endorphins in response to alcohol.

That is a biological trait—like blue eyes or brown hair. You are born that way, and you can never change it. That is why people with the condition must never drink.

"Some people begin treatment thinking they can improve by simply drinking less. That can't be the case if they are dependent. Because whenever anything is excessively pleasurable it is addictive. When someone who is dependent drinks, it is Heaven He has a great cascade of endorphins that is released in the hypothalamus and received and interpreted in the cortex as intense pleasure, security and freedom from pain. If you have ever broken a leg or an arm, you might have noticed that it didn't hurt when it first happened: you felt no pain . That's because of the release of endorphins.

"How many people in this country do you think of this condition?

"About 50 percent."

"Well no, that's high. It's about one in seven were 15 percent. In some groups it is higher much higher—Native Americans, for example. And that's further evidence that the condition is genetic."

"When the other people drink, the six out of seven, it's pleasurable. It's nice, but it's not Heaven. They can take it or leave it. And again that's the essence of dependence. Whenever anything is Heaven, it's irresistible and its addictive.

"That applies to all people and to all advanced animals. That was actually shown inadvertently in the lab in the late 1950s. They were mapping the brain by planting electrodes in various parts and watching the animal's response. They used cats for these experiments. They found an area in the hypothalamus, part of the base of the brain, that they called the pleasure center because when it was stimulated, the cat behaved as though he was getting intense pleasure, like a been dropped in a field of catnip. They attach the wires from the electrodes to a big red button included in front of the cat so that he could press it with his paw. What do you think the cat did all day?"

"Press the red button."

"Right. And although it wasn't realized then, here was a ready made model of addiction. The key was unhindered access to pleasure. That is, the excess of endorphins made repetition of the behavior irresistible and that applies to all people regardless of intelligence, income or morality and to all advanced animals. If a behavior or substance gives excess endorphin production in a certain individual, it is addictive for that individual. (The ability to release excess endorphins doesn't develop until a person is in his very late teens or early '20s. In fact the human brain grows until about the age of 25. That is why children are not addictable. Their brains have not matured to the point that they can produce excess endorphin.)

"It's typical of several neurological disorders that they are both hereditary and develop only at a certain age. Huntington's Chorea is the classic example. People with this disorder cannot stop writhing. They move their arms and feet in an undue lading riding motion and the look is though they're dancing, but they can't stop, though they do everything to mask the movement and make it look like something else. Alcohol dependence is like that and if you have it, there is nothing you can do to change it. Children have a 50 percent chance of getting it if one parent has a. They wouldn't hear that until their about 50 when it declares itself and they know one way or the other.

"Parkinson's disease is like that. It declares itself around 55 to 60 years of age. It can also be caused by damage, accidents, substances, medicines, or other biological conditions but in its pure form that's what it is.

"Schizophrenia is also such a condition, again poorly recognized, that it declares itself in a broader range between 20 and 40 years. (Probably it is actually a group of similar conditions that declare themselves at different times in the range.)

"In any case it is a peculiar ready of neurological conditions that they are like a time bomb waiting to go off. Most medical conditions are not like that. The reason that alcohol dependence does not develop earlier is that the brain simply is not mature enough to generate a sufficiently large cascade of endorphin until around age 20. That is why children did not develop dependency but young adults do. The brain continues to grow into one's mid twenties. And undergoes constant change as one ages and learns. It is truly, simultaneously, the most constant, unchanging and rigid organ and at the same time the most flexible and rapidly adaptive. (It depends on what level of structure one talks about.)

"Alcohol is dangerous to the brain and other tissues because it is a solvent for fats. The cell wall, especially that of brain cells, is made mostly of fat molecules. Proteins and carbohydrates are embedded in and attached to the wall of fat molecules. Alcohol, like anesthetics, loosens up the structure of the cell wall, in some case dissolves the cell wall so that the cell bursts open, like a soap bubble. More often the cell is not killed, but it loses structure. Particularly, dendrites are lopped off, or dissolved off the cell body. Dendrites are like branches on a tree. They're literally as complex and intricate; and the brain is like a thick forest where each tree intermingles with its neighbor. When one drinks or takes other substances that destroy cell structure it is like thinning the forest. The longer one drinks the thinner the forest, the less complex one's thoughts become. And if you know someone who has continued to drink you can see that increasing simplicity; the collaterals that his thoughts can take become fewer and narrower.

"The good news is that if one stops drinking and nurtures the brain adequately the dendrites will regrow and intellect and mood will recover. Also learning probably stimulates and represents growth of dendritic pathways; and some antidepressants may further stimulate growth or regrowth of dendritic branches. Intelligence, more properly, some part of intelligence is probably dependent on dendritic density. (Certainly there are other chemical and genetic factors.)

"Not everything that is addictive is as destructive as alcohol—nicotine for example, or caffeine. The popular benzodiazepines are very similar to alcohol pharmacologically and easily as destructive to the cell membrane as alcohol. Keeping someone on Valium or one of its dozen cousins three times a day is akin to recommending a shot of whiskey three times a day.

"Stimulants such as amphetamines (such as cocaine—crack or powder) are also very destructive if for no other reason than causing spasms of the small muscle-walled arterioles. When blood is agitated, it clots, thereby occluding blood flow and causing many (often undectable) strokes—the same mechanism but on a smaller scale by which they can cause heart attacks in otherwise healthy people.

"By the way, did you want Antabuse?"

Chapter 4—What's to Decide?

Berghman the fat jovial (when he wasn't grouchy) child psychiatrist, puffed out, red faced, joked to me. We were neck to neck in the fat race; really I think he was substantially more rotund, ruddy, and plethoric; but he joked that it was for us. I didn't seriously consider it.

It took me about six months. My blood sugar stayed up, my weight didn't go down.

My chunky, chunky patient described her failing marriage to me. I referred her for gastric reduction.

"No. He's not going to pay any of the credit cards. He has to pay $60 rent off post, and he considers that fair."

"How much are they?"

"Fifteen and twenty dollars a month. And he's unhappy about the operation. He says that will take a year longer."

"A year longer? How does he figure that?"

"He thinks it will be six months before I am able to work again."

"That shouldn't be. They say allow six weeks after the operation. So you do want the operation?"

"I don't see an alternative. I'm five foot two and weigh about 260 pounds. My mother's diabetes was so bad that she needed both feet amputated; and she was miserable all the time. I know that will happen to me. Also she was about my age when her diabetes started ."

"You haven't heard from the surgeons yet?"

"No."

"Well let's submit the consult again and they'll set you up with the surgeons for an appointment. Armstrong and Chung are the guys that do it here. You know we have to get a time before you lose your benefits. On the outside this operation costs from 30 to 40 thousand dollars. It's amazing any insurance company supports it. It must be that it is reasonably effective and that it is cheaper than the complications of obesity.

"But to make sure I've justified the consult so they can't turn us down, tell me about your previous dieting. I assume you've done that."

"Yes, in fact, I have. I was president of TOPS last year."

"President? And how much weight did you lose in that year?"

"None. I gained 60 pounds. I may go back and tell them it isn't working."

"60 pounds. That's interesting. Now TOPS is based on an addictive model."

"Yes, it's a 12 step program."

"And the group support is an essential factor.... I wonder why it doesn't work? You see I don't think it's an addiction—obesity is something else. And it's right to concentrate on the stomach, not on the brain.

"The difference is that eating has to do with satiety, and satiety ultimately is a form of discomfort. And nobody eats when they are uncomfortably full or when they feel too full to eat another bite. It actually hurts. It's one of the most uncomfortable feelings we regularly go through.

"Now with drinking or marijuana use or cocaine use there is really no satiety. There are debilitating states that keep the person from using anymore at that time—unconsciousness or continual vomiting—but unconsciousness is not a state of mind like satiety.

"There are more and more people becoming heavy in this country and if it's a disease or an addiction, then it's an epidemic. It doesn't make sense. Dependencies are inherited conditions; and while there do appear to be heritable factors in obesity, these do not appear determinate The closest similarity might be to a substance such as cocaine that is so effective in releasing endorphins that some people regard them as nearly universally addictive. Some of that thought is based on animal studies. I don't think it's the case, however with a free human population. I predict that most people if they have unlimited access to cocaine would not choose to use it even regularly or infrequently—would not in fact even abuse it. A minority would abuse it and a smaller minority would be dependent.

"Then we do the problem great injustice to assume that everyone who is overweight is addicted to food. It's just not the case and I predict we will not be able to get a good response working with the addiction model. (However the converse of the argument may also be true that some people are truly dependent on food.)

"The truth is that given the amount of food in our country, the availability of it, and the affordability of it, over eating for many people is a normal behavior. The availability of food in our country and the decreased amount of exertion necessary to earn it are unprecedented in the entire history of the world. People may be starving elsewhere, and just 50 years ago Stalin was starving 40 million people, and it was easy; there wasn't enough food and it saved his shooting twenty million people. But those are far away dreams to most Americans. 100 years ago in this country the necessity of providing food and earning it kept nearly everyone busy every day. If you worked on a farm you weren't fat. Also a much larger per cent of income went to food. And eating was much more ritualistic and much more important as it is in Europe still. The further you go back in history the more difficult food was to come by. That's why easily grown food like the potato was such a boon.

"But now unexpectedly, miraculously, even unpredictably the situation has changed. Consider that until a few hundred years ago it was eat and run, catch as catch can. That's what the stomach's about. If you had food today you were lucky. You might eat tomorrow, you might not. It might be two or three days before you ate again. You had to take as much as you could while it was available. You had to stuff it and store it. And that's what the stomach's about; its for storage. It's to take what you couldn't use now, along with you. Typically predators use the stomach that way . They devour their kill, take it to a safer place, and disgorge it to be eaten later in peace. (That gorging and disgorging behavior may even be an origin bulimia.)

"Nowadays food is sold on every corner in myriad varieties. At home we store it in the ice box and in the cupboards. We keep it in the car. We bring it to the office. We don't have a kill that will spoil or be stolen if we don't take our fill now. We don't have Pharaohs, kings, dictators or other tyrants who will dole it out in homeopathic quantities.

"The stomach is outmoded obsolete, defunct; it is no longer necessary and the behavior associated with it is also anachronism . The storage function of the stomach has been replaced by an elaborate technology. Consider also that it doesn't take many calories a day to gain weight. Many people gain weight slowly, insidiously. A hundred calories a day excess such as from a bottle of soda would be about 3000 calories a month. That translates into a pound of weight gain; and in a year to 12 pounds. After five years it's 60 pounds and after ten years, a hundred twenty pounds. Amazingly, the claim of some very heavy people that "I don't really eat that much" may therefore be true.

"From that perspective, gastric reduction makes a good deal of sense. Satiety is still the key. People stop eating when their stomachs are full. The sensation of fullness is what brings eating to cessation, given the availability of food. A smaller stomach leads much more quickly to satiety. And satiety leads to a cessation of eating, and eating less leads to decreased intake which, even if only a hundred calories a day, leads to weight loss.

"Linus Pauling made a similar argument very convincingly, about vitamin C. His point was that we used to get a lot more of it, before we started cultivating grains or eating greater amounts of fish and meat.

We used to eat many more fresh green leaves, maybe a hundred thousand years ago; and we have not yet evolved out of that need for great quantities of exogenous vitamin C. "

Chapter 5—DOING IT

Getting the Suburban ready. Old diesel smelling thing. The bed? We need a bed with it? I thought I'd sleep on some quilts. No you're right. We'll put a mattress in. It's loaded so fully. Will there be room?

Everyone has to come. My three boys included. My oldest has to leave his parrot behind. My brother couldn't clear enough time to watch them. The old car runs smoothly. It was much too expensive to rent and we put the money instead into repairs on the old diesel Suburban—a fuel leak, new rear shocks, oil change, new starter, ignition switch.

Up the 95. South Carolina. Looks like its swamp 50 miles inward. Haven't been here since I was 12 and we stopped at some little house run by a svelte Miss

Pickles long ago. Further up the 95. We're delighted to see the name Francis Marion everywhere, even the Francis Marion Motel. Gets us talking about the Swamp Fox, singing the Swamp Fox song and talking about vinegar and water.

The trip is fine until around 5:30 as it darkens. Heavy cold rain; the wipers fail. Knew it would be something on the old thing. We stop at a motel at the next exit and my children are delighted to be there. That night we watch an old Disney story about geese.

The next morning is clear and we complete the 50 miles to Richmond. It's cold up here. Refreshing— almost a northern town. We scout out the hospital. Many buildings over a hundred years old. Can still see the Civil War here: the old train station, the old factories and town houses—treasures well preserved. We scout out the hospital. It's a cute little large town. Again history everywhere: the old Confederate capital. Some other monstrosity of an old stone building.

Are these my last thoughts before I leave my children—to what—am I right to do it? I still have choices…choices…choices overrated.

The area around the hospital has that large town feel—nothing compared to the places where I trained, in size and intimidation. It's cute, comfortable, just threatening and serious enough. Nice old brick buildings to live in. A place like this, that's so comfortable is where I'd like my sons to go to medical school. We know how to get there—to what they call simply Main Hospital (9th floor conference room tomorrow).

Now for breakfast. We head back down the 95 and find a place called Sarah's Pancake House—a chain up here. Great atmosphere. Looks like it was built during the Civil War or in Colonial times; the two histories mingle here. I order a large breakfast—a skillet with hash browns, hash and fried eggs. Service is glacial.

Next for a place to stay that isn't downtown, but has reasonably quick access. I guessed straight north on the outer belt, and there's nothing there. We continue east on it until we get near the airport.

We find a place called the Microtel with kitchenettes in every room, and they give us a weekly rate. One of the adjoining rooms is for the disabled. No indoor pool, but we can't manage everything.

The next day at 10:00, the 9th floor conference room. We park in the large ominous garage and go up the long, covered gang way to the main hospital. It's cold and winter here—just as it was in medical school in Cleveland—like being at Metro General only smaller, cleaner, cuter.

We find the conference room and peer in the little window—a few minutes early. The surgeons are seated around Dr. Sugerman. He's obviously the head of the department. He looks up and sees my face;

we're a few minutes early. We understand each other. Now a few more patients gather quietly, heavily.

The door opens and the surgeons walk out hurriedly. Sugerman stops only briefly facing us saying blandly, "Hello…Everybody." It's a large metropolitan hospital— the county hospital—have I made the right decision?

A somewhat heavy, pregnant nurse with long chestnut hair comes along and leads us into the room. Soon a very thin reserved nurse in pants and jacket suit fastidiously groomed joins her and we all sit down. Some of these people weigh four hundred pounds. They are quiet and sweet mannered.

The nurse says, " Sir, excuse me. Could we ask you to sit over here?" pointing across the room. "We have to bring in a chair for a patient." They clear the single chairs away and bring in a simple two seater couch. Here comes William. He must weigh four hundred fifty pounds. He's a kid—late teens, early '20s, a pleasant disposition—wearing a baseball cap back-wards. His left leg is wrapped repeatedly with gauze and he seems somehow in pain simply to be so heavy; walking doesn't look comfortable; sitting doesn't look comfortable; poor William.

The lecture begins. I'm so and so. I'm the nurse for this project; I've been doing it for years, and I'll be delivering soon; so, so and so here, who is so slim and proper in the fancy clothes, will be doing the program for me. She reviews the procedure, the dietary restric-tions, what it's like handling a midline incision, what to expect after surgery—who will go straight to the ICU afterward: those with asthma, those with compli-cations, those with sleep apnea, those who are extremely heavy, those who smoked until a month ago, those who'll need drainage tubes.

If you've had bypass surgery before, you'll need a gas-trostomy tube (G-tube) in the lower part of your stomach to keep it from distending. Everybody gets an NG tube and a foley catheter. She talks about patient controlled anesthesia (press the button as often as you like) about activity—how it decreases pneumonia and deadly blood clots, and improves weight loss. You'll be up the day of surgery. Keep the head of your bed elevated, to keep pressure off the incision and help with breathing. Compression hose will squeeze your legs to prevent clots. Use your incentive inspirometer to keep your lungs clear.

On the third day after surgery, an upper GI with gastropaque is done, and if suture lines are tight, a barium shake follows. Jill, the heavy nurse warns us it will be uncomfortable because of the cold x-ray table and the fullness. She says it will feel impossible to finish the barium shake.

You go home after the seventy two hours approved by insurance. To avoid a ventral (abdominal) hernia you must, for one month, not lift more than ten pounds; avoid holding babies, children or animals; avoid heavy house work, avoid sexual intercourse. You may drive again after two weeks.

All of these are true if you have the usual incision from breast bone to belly button. Some surgeons are doing laporoscopic gastric reductions and that procedure should simplify aftercare, decreasing change to muscle and skin caused by scarring, and also be aesthetically superior. Currently many of the midline scars are revised a year after the procedure, simultaneous to a "tummy tuck" that is done to draw up the excess floppy skin. Still, if possible, the inevitable weakening of the abdominal wall caused by the midline incision is best avoided. Conversely data is not in on the laporoscopic procedure. That is, we do not know that it is as safe and as effective. Eventually as skill and technology improve that would expectedly be the case.

Another thing to think about is the gallbladder. If it's diseased or has stones and removal is indicated, your surgeon will. Some surgeons remove the gallbladder during the procedure regardless. That is because the rapid weight loss, caused by breakdown of body fat, will give you gallstones. Dr. Sugerman prefers to leave the gallbladder and use medicine called Actigall for six months to prevent the development of gallstones, during the period of greatest weight loss.

She talks about the incision line and advises a shower every day and patting the staples dry as the best way to keep everything clean. (I prefer to keep mine dry and use Betadine on the incision every day. I had good results doing so.) Watch for redness, swelling, or heat at the incision, soreness or pain at the incision, drainage from the incision, or temperature over one hundred. These might indicate infection. The same observations apply to the exit site of the G. tube.

You must avoid pregnancy for one year after surgery. Pregnancy is very dangerous for mother and child and could result in birth defects. Also rapid weight loss increases fertility so that you must be extra careful.

You may experience some depression. It is usually easily handled and is a normal sequel of major surgery. There is no contra indication to the use of anti-depressants such as Prozac or Zoloft.

You will have to take a multi-vitamin, calcium, and B12 on an ongoing basis for the rest of your life. Menstruating women will need to take iron. Supplemental B12 is necessary because intrinsic factor which allows its absorption is found only in the lower part of the stomach—the part that is now blocked from receiving nutrients. Calcium and are iron are also best absorbed there. Failure to take adequate B12 can over years lead to a form of dementia called Wernecke's Encephalopathy—again easy to prevent.

To me these are not burdensome requirements. Everyone should take supplemental vitamins anyway, especially considering the American diet. (Read those nutrition labels and weep.)

Another restriction after the procedure is not to take any nonsteroidal anti-inflammatories. These are the aspirin type drugs including aspirin, Advil, Motrin, Alieve, Excedrin, B.C. powders and Peptobismal. They greatly increase the risk for ulcer. I am distressed at that, as I'm a firm believer in an aspirin a day. Dr. Sugerman says you may be able to take these medications along with Cytotec—a prescription antiulcer medicine; and I'll have to explore that possibility; that is, two pills instead of one.

Vomiting may be caused by eating too fast, too much, or eating the wrong food; or sometimes drinking fluid with meals. Most patients will at some point vomit.

Stomal stenosis is a tightening, or stricture at the opening between the stomach and intestine. It usually manifests about four weeks after surgery. The main symptom is vomiting after eating, sometimes even after drinking. It is usually easily treated with outpatient endoscopy, but should be done as soon as possible.

As the procedure is an extreme assault on the stomach and instestine, involves sututre lines, and healing surfaces, ulcers are an increased possibility. The symptoms are severe nausea or pain with eating.

You may also experience a change in bowel habits, either constipation, loose stool or gas. These are dealt with in the usual ways. Also you'll need a yearly check up with your surgeon's office.

These are the rates of complications in the Medical College of Virginia's series:

Major wound infection	2.7%
Incisional hernia	25.0%
Stomal Stenosis	16.0%
Ulcer at the hook up	13.0%
Gallstones	
without anti-gallstone med	33.0%
with Actigall	2.0%
Blood Clots in	
veins or lungs	0.5%
Leak (intra-abdominal	
abscess or peritonitis)	1.5%
Death within 30 days	0.5%

Now for the diet—the nurses' favorite part. You must follow some simple rules. Keep in mind, you must work with it. It can be beaten either by over expanding your pouch, or by eating the wrong foods too frequently. Among sweets the following must be avoided:

Cake	Molasses
Cookies	Pastries
Candy	Pies
Chewing gum	Pudding
Custard	Sugary Cereals
Granola	Sweet Rolls
Honey	Condensed Milk
Ice cream	Sweetened Fruit
Jam/Jelly	Syrup

Do not drink:

Regular Sodas	Gatorade
Regular Fruit Drinks	Ultra Slim Fast
Sweetened Seltzers	Or any sweetened
Ensure	beverage, unless
	with saccharin or
	aspartame

You must avoid food with added sugar or high-fat. (That advice would be hollow were it not for the peculiar change in appetite and preferences that occurs after the procedure.) It sounds hard, but it won't be. Avoid :

Corn chips	Onion rings
Nabs	Peanuts
Microwave popcorn	Pork Rinds
Doritos	Potato chips
Fritos	Anything cooked
Cheetos	in lard, bacon fat,
Regular fast food	Crisco, or
Fried Food	margarine

Use butter substitutes.

Eating sweets can cause "dumping" syndrome, characterized by severe diarrhea, nausea, light headedness, and stomach cramps.

Determining what has added sugar can be tricky. The problem mostly comes with processed foods, and fortunately nutrition labels can help. If you see any of the following sugars in the first three ingredients do not eat that food:

Brown sugar

Confectioner's sugar

Corn syrup

Corn sweeteners

Dextrose

Fructose

Fruit sugar

Glucose

Granulated sugar

Honey

Invert sugar

Lactose

Laevulose

Maltose

Mannitol

Maple syrup

Molasses

Raw sugar

Sorbitol

Sorghum

Sucrose

Turbinado sugar

Xylitol

Do not be fooled by the grams of sugar on the Nutrition Facts label. That number includes both natural sugars (such as those found in milk or fruit—acceptable—and added sugars—as in the list above). No matter what that number is, you need only avoid those foods that have sugar listed as one of the first three ingredients.

Products with NutraSweet and Saccharin are fine. But it is important not to fill up on diet products, because your appetite (and stomach) will be much smaller. And you must get adequate protein every day. If you don't, you'll lose muscle, and your hair will fall out. Females need 50 grams of protein, and males around 63 grams. In the first month, because your diet must be pureed or otherwise soft, getting enough protein can be a challenge. Generally milk and yogurt have about eight grams of protein per cup. Cottage cheese is a surprising bargain with a whopping 26 grams of protein per cup. Also protein shakes used by body builders are a boon as they generally have anywhere from 15 to 50 grams of protein per ounce of powder. One ounce of these will dissolve in a cup of milk but trying to concentrate it further to increase protein intake may cause it to clump. Peanut butter is not a good source of protein because of its high-fat content. Beans in every form and various vegetable burgers are also a helpful source of protein. (You may need Lactaid or other gas aids such as Beano.)

Meat, eggs, seafood, and poultry are also just fine, but it's hard to find palatable ways to blenderize them during the first month. Powdered skim milk is also a useful adjunct for increasing protein (about eight grams for every 1/3 cup of powder).

The dietician entered the room and showed some simple diets for a day. These required:

Six proteins

Three fats

Two starches

Two fruits

Two vegetables

Every day.

That's the substance of the meeting. But the people who came to the meeting are more important. I found them to be lovely people. They're all at least a hundred to a hundred fifty pounds heavier than I. But they are sweet hearts. Not being so sweet myself I almost feel an outsider. They have a gentleness, an affability, an all accepting nature—sweet hearts, smiling fat Buddhas—that gives the room a warmth peculiar among strangers. We understand already some important things about each other—the stigma, the pain, the ostracism, the hopelessness, the knowledge one can never lose weight on one's own. Soon that ordeal may be over. Even good health may be around the corner—something we have faked but never known.

Remember William? He's still sitting there, fat and affable as ever. But where can William go without astounding people, and therefore becoming the object of their overflowing mental energy? When the pregnant nurse, Jill, talks about no sex for a month, she pauses for a moment, stating that usually someone makes a witty comment. Nobody does, but William shows disappointment and makes a plaintive noise. I say to myself, "Come on William what kind of sex could you have known? Is anything accessible to you?" And you can't help but empathize with him fully.

Another enormous girl in a nice green dress, later that day taps me on the shoulder, as we wait (interminably) to have our blood drawn—almost flirtatiously.

And before the chest x-ray (part of the pre-op) I'm waiting with an old boy very round about the middle, who tells me about his mother and how Dr. Sugerman is the best. And when Sugerman was about to bypass his mother he found cancer in her gallbladder. He didn't proceed and she lived six months after. I can't describe the tenderness with which he conveyed the story. Clearly he loved his mother very much. He was a sweetheart. And clearly all these people were capable of great love and affection. How sad that the world abused them and turned them away as freaks or unworthies. (Conversely, how strange the Orientals could so freely embrace the chubby Buddha. Could we accept a tubby Christ?)

I'm a psychiatrist, and I consider the intellectual side of psychiatry a foolish romp into the desert. (That is, Sophocles is smarter than Freud any day.) But one thing about psychiatry is that you get to know people quickly—after listening to thousands, your ears sharpen. And I have never met at once such an all-accepting little group of people. Clearly these are people who were very close to a loving, nurturing mother. How wonderful that love must have been. (I know it was in my case, and I hope I'm not projecting.) They accepted the whole world with an acceptance resembling that they originally knew and gave. They would devour the whole world because (despite its hurt to them) they love it, and they anticipate it will love them. Of course, one can only devour the whole world for so long, before getting in trouble. How interesting that the surgeon who cares or knows so little what these people feel can cure them. How interesting to find a surgical cure for a psychiatric problem. Beats lobotomy by a long shot.

The rest of the day is spent eternally waiting for labs and then having a fatuous conversation with an anesthesiologist. If you can, you may want to consider avoiding county hospitals, teaching hospitals, and other places with interns and residents. Remember they're there to learn, or as Curly says <u>practice.</u>

Chapter 6—Darkest Hour

It's 2:00. The room is dark. I'm awake. Where and why? Oh yes. It's the day of surgery. I don't want to be awake. I want to be as little conscious as possible. I won't get back to sleep now. I could still escape. I might not make it. No, I must go, because my sugar is up and I won't be around, to help my boys. If I don't go ahead. If I don't do it. That would be rum— to leave Sugerman in the lurch: "No, the patient changed his mind at the last moment."

It is a cold and lonely place to be. There is no return and it will be Hell waking up. But I'll be on the other side. But I could be orphaning my children. No I'll survive. God told me so. Trust in Him.

I remembered now the evening before. I had steak and potato, as the nurse had said to eat heavily but be NPO past midnight. We went to the grocery to get Pepcid as the anesthesiologist had said. We had fun goofing around in the grocery. While I was waiting in the Suburban I very gently backed into some guy in his little sedan. It was a source of endless merriment as the guy waited a minute, then burst out of his car, yelling, " Oh my car, my car! I've got to see your insurance card! I've got to see your insurance card!"

I phlegmatically rub the back of his bumper and can't find a dent or scratch. He sees that's the case and suddenly reverses himself, "Oh that's ok man, that's ok man, that's ok." and hops back into his car. I have the encounter endlessly reenacted to me, to my children's oedipal delight.

But that was last night. Now it's two o'clock. I get about two more hours or sleep. We wake up at five, and my family drop me off. They will return to the motel and sleep while I do the procedure: I would not think of keeping them up so early on such a day. But I will not take a cab. I want to kiss them just before I die, and not be in the cold purgatory of a stranger's indifference. I kiss them all.

I report to Ward 9A. They direct me to a hospital room and a none too friendly black woman gives me a gown and some socks with rubber skids on them, and instructs me to put my stuff in a plastic bag. I sit in my robe and "slippers" calmly waiting. Eventually she leads me toward another patient's room, but he needs a minute or two. I hear his preacher saying a prayer with him, and can even share some of it as I stand outside in the hallway.

He comes out—a thin gray haired fellow—in his '50s. A man in his early 30s in a gray suit, glasses and a mustache and long hair stands outside his door. I imagined he's a step son. He says "Andrew." And they embrace and he turns down the hallway. The phlegmatic black woman leads us to the row of ominous silver doored elevators and he comments, "It's like being led to the gas chamber, isn't it?" "Yeah," I say, "It's like something from your dreams." He makes me think of the father or my best friend in high school—William Linn, the good carpenter. Down to the cold basement. A small part of the ramus of his right jaw has been removed. We're led to two rows of beds, about four in each line. He takes the bed opposite me, a nurse draws the silky white curtain, and that is the last I see of him.

Chapter 7—Waking

I wake up around twelve. I think it is.

It's a nightmare. I feel paralyzed. I can barely breath. I have a horrible blow-by mask over my mouth. (I hate these things; they always give them to you when you're suffocating.) But at least the air feels cool and moist, and I can suck some of it in, but just barely. It feels good because I feel hot and dry, and so uncomfortable I can barely stand it. I can't move. That's what drives me crazy. My lower back feels hot and sore and sweaty (the bed has a plastic cover). But I can't move, and my throat is incredibly sore and dry, and I don't know why. (I have an NG tube down my left nostril.) I hear the suction running, but can't see the dark red blood collecting there. But the worst of the nightmare is the paralysis. I can move my head, but I feel as though I can't move any of the rest of my body. Actually I try , and try, and I can, but just barely. It proves to me I'm not paralyzed. But I'm so weak. You haven't experienced a nightmare until you've experienced paralysis or something like it, and my heart goes out to those who have.

Worst of all, there is no one in the room. I can't ask someone to move me from this torturous position.

Strangest of all are these balloons that inflate and then suddenly deflate. They start in your ankles and inflate progressively up the legs, squeezing all the way. Kinky. I'm amazed I know what it's for. When I was a resident we had only pressure hose. I think to myself, "That's terrific. You can't get a DVT or a PE with something like that!" It exerts more pressure on the veins than walking. It really squeezes in fast, and at this point, feels both good and bad, and just plain weird—but I'm glad to have them. (The one fatality I've heard of was a nephew of one of my older patients, about my age, 46, who died of pulmonary emboli—clots that usually form in the legs and migrating to the lungs cause severe sometimes fatal pulmonary distress.) No doubt he didn't have leggings like these—povero.

Then in a flash, I realize I've made it. I'm alive. I've done it. I've walked through the fire and come out on the other end.

I have years of living ahead—years with my children. I'm going to make it! Somehow the thought gives me the patience to bear it, and I decide to suck in the cool moist air, like a soothing drug, and soon fall asleep.

CHAPTER 8—DAYS TO ENDURE

I had many other adventures in my three days in the hospital. They're not perfectly relevant, but I'll sum them up to give you an idea of what you might encounter. And again, I do not want to dissuade you from the procedure. I believe in the procedure. I just want you to be prepared. You may skip this chapter: it has very little to do with gastric reduction. It was a difficult three days. I'd summarize as follows:

The Adventure of the Kinked Foley—
or the How Much Can Your Bladder Hold Game

Cup of Crushed Ice and Foam Swabs—
Greatest Pleasure Known to Man

Up and Walking the First Day

Wife and Boys Visit—Gratia Deo

Stay Up Most of the Night—VS's etc—
Adventures with Kim and Shirley

Fun Roommate Number One—
Who Runs Marathons but Has Colon Cancer—
He Doesn't Know What Stage.

Young black male with a colostomy he doesn't know how to manage and whose German girlfriend won't shut up about Campbell's Cream of Mushroom Soup and Mc Donald's Fish Sandwich. Unnecessary admit. taken fastidious care of by Phillipino resident who would have done better to run down to the ER himself and have screened this one out. Watches TV literally interminably. Leaves plastic quart container half full of poop in bathroom; thinks nurses told him to save it. What steams me most about this character is that he enjoys it here; he's a professional patient. He loves being waited on. He keeps asking for "a cup of that chicken broth."

NG Tube Out

Forgive me for screaming—seems to be a personal insult to the resident.

More Crushed Ice and Swabs

Sit up in Chair

Walk Round and Round the Ward with IV Pole

Wife and Boys Visit

Fun Roommate Number Two

Middle aged alcoholic black male—dubbed Suction Man by my children—who arrives with a suction tube in his mouth, making a ghostly slushy, vacuum sound.

He immediately turns on the TV and continues interminably to suction himself. I expect to see tentacles under the curtain that divides us. Mercifully, the nurse tells him Dr Pippin has just been paged, and he's turning around on the highway right now. The Hand of God! Pippin arrives and tells Suction Man he's bleeding way too much after his tonsillectomy, and he'll have to whisk him off to surgery. Suction Man can't speak, but groans as he suctions.

I say a little prayer of thanks, and ponder how the Lord provides for his children: "Thou preparest a table before me in the midst of mine enemies." I'm exhausted. I need to heal. Now I can sleep until three or four when they roll this guy back in, still suctioning, no doubt. Sure enough: 0300 and the Suction's back! I'm awake! But…I got my sleep—Ha! Sure, go ahead, take my vitals! He's back watching TV. I'll sit in my chair a bit. Then I'll take a walk and amaze everyone at four in the morning. Yes, could I have the ice chips and the swabs—we celebrate every little victory.

Round and Round with the IV Pole

Adventures with Colleen

who thinks at one point I'm keeling over, and amazingly, is able to get her arms around my entire belly to prop me up. Blissfully, Suction falls asleep, and I turn the TV off to make sure the miracle is real. Sleep for three hours. Residents march in. The leader must be an orthopod, to judge by his brusque, loud, athletic approach. He removes the bandage, and one of his henchmen removes the foley. I scream.

Suction man's up watching the morning talk shows. Colleen asks who she can call to pick him up. He rasps out her name—a long lost girlfriend. She doesn't even know he's here. Colleen calls. She comes. A touching reunion after many months. She will bring him home and take care of him, amidst lush violins.

Meanwhile, back in reality, I can't urinate. At last Suction Man and the Sucker are gone in a sentimental blur, Colleen the enchanted audience.

Wife and children visit. Running out of things to do in Richmond, without spending too much. They'll go to the Science Museum and to a giant bookstore. My wife's the cheapest woman in the world. She warned me we'd be stuck with a huge bill for any procedure that costs 25 to 40 thousand dollars. (She was wrong.) Betya anything she won't spend more than fifty dollars today.

Now for the first time, my eldest, in moving my gown, catches a glimpse of my incision, irregular, overlapping, with large staples at uneven intervals. It is a shocking sight to a loving son and my heart fills with joy when I see how intelligently he handles his response. First he sees and understands at a glance. He shows that little shock of unpleasant recognition, betrayed by a start in every muscle: that shows intelligence and sensitivity. He quickly suppresses his own reaction and damps the start before its completion. That's further evidence of good judgment, caution, intelligence, sensitivity, and politeness. I feel a flush of pride in him, his brothers, and the job his mother has done in educating them. How sensible and noble for a twelve year old.

Nurse comes in and tells me how to take a sponge bath. (Thanks, I needed that. In a private hospital they'd bathe and massage you, lazy thing.)

Down to the basement for radiology—gastrograffin and barium—to make sure there aren't any leaks. Held up on the way by Stacie, know it all nurse, who wants to postpone the studies for a pulse of 106 because Fernandez (I occasionally see him skulking about) ordered a stat EKG an hour ago. I protest to the infuriatingly bland nurse (the one who helped Jill) and at last we go down. The radiology staff are competent and kind. The study is fine and painless. Sugerman agrees with me, "That's ridiculous!" he says, with a bit too much affect, especially for him. (Once you get off a radiology schedule, it's twelve hours before you get back on. So far so good.)

I still can't urinate because of the pain. Up and pushing the IV pole around. Some resident jokes to me, "Lap 20!" The goofy student reminds me there is an incidence of UTI (urinary tract infection) of 10% per day, and I complain to my favorite resident, Dumont, that my urethral meatus is so sore I can't go, and could they send me up some viscous lidocaine. That takes at least four and a half hours and in the meantime, the evil resident from the Philippines threatens to straight cath me if I don't urinate. There's not enough room in this town for the both of us!

Fun Roommate Number Three

dubbed Hispanuola by my children—some young Spanish guy who comes in with two older people, and for some reason, I have trouble figuring out the relationship between them. He tells the nurse in his weakened, broken English, that his name is Fernando Montoya Antonio Perez de Cuillhar. She marvels at the length of his name. He's been in a car wreck. He has no apparent injuries. The nurse asks him if he was wearing his seat belt. Yes, he says. So it must be a seat belt or steering wheel trauma, and he must be admitted to rule out further chest injury such as expanding mediastinum—a tear in aorta or vena cava from sudden acceleration. He sounds feeble, and the older people, who treat him as a child must be his parents, even though he is twenty four. He puts the TV on while they visit, and keeps it on even when he falls asleep at eleven.

The lidocaine comes. The resident Matthew Dumont hands it to me—the whole four-ounce tube of it, and says, "Apply liberally." I can urinate with great difficulty, using gobs of it. I pass first gas explosively.

Up and walking again; vitals; insulin. First explosion post MOM, kindly given by Tricia. She's been obsequious since my return from radiology, but now she has her revenge. A shower. I pull my IV because it looks inflamed. Blood all over 'til I lift my hand above my heart. (Infected IVs are a major cause of nosocomial infections.)

Adventures with Renee

For some reason that's a major problem. I feel embarrassment for her as she doesn't know the first thing about starting an IV and can't admit it. But she's being brave and she'll try; and I'm being brave, and I'll let her. (She likes the way the underside of my arm ripples when I repeatedly make a fist, and she says, "You've got it going on the other side of your arm." which confirms my notion she won't be able to start it.) She tells me her ex retired from the army. And after two or three times says she thinks she can't get it because she's intimidated by me. She calls the student, who is somewhat arrogant, somewhat likeable mostly defensive and utterly unpracticed in starting IVs. Is this a hospital or what? He says he wouldn't mind trying two times more if I were anesthetized. (That reminds me of the six inexplicable pin pricks right through the tendon bundles of my left wrist— misguided attempts at ABG's while I was under.) Fortunately Renee knows Diane, who never misses. And she doesn't. Blessed Diane.

Now I won't dry up overnight. Out for a walk. Up in the chair. Children visit. Hispanuola falls asleep; leaves TV on that I promptly nix . He snores heavily the whole night; and it is the most peaceful night I've had.

Next morning is Saturday. Hispanuola's up watching five torturous hours of new smart aleck Disney cartoons. Later, lusting for comedy he switches to the House on CNN and I get to hear those dramatic historical moments when Bob Livingston resigns.

They deliver the test juice—six little 20cc cups. As it's brought in, Hispanuola (I swear to God) starts moaning, "Fooood, fooood." I chuckle to myself: If only he knew what it was. His little brother visits with his parents. The child talks excitedly about what they can do after they sue the other driver. So that's it! That's why he's playing such a hurting, illiterate, sad sack.

Twenty four hours after admission, Hispanuola's ready to check out. At last he gets fooood—a chicken salad sandwich—and takes a shower. The nurse, lisping, ambling Melissa, tells me the person he hit died. Hispanuola walked away unscathed. She also tells me he marked Spanish on the admission sheet, as the only language he speaks. His English is perfect. Angling for that suit money no doubt.

Soon after the test juices, comes the test meal: pureed spinach, pureed chicken—stuck together as some kind of loaf—tomato soup, and milk. I eat it all, and think I'll burst.

Then Sugerman calls and says,"I'm playing hooky"

That's fine," I say, "You deserve to." He asks me how the meal was, and says if I don't die, I can go home in three hours.

CHAPTER 9—WHAT'S IT LIKE?

It's amazing. It hurts for weeks, and you keep wondering, is everything ok? It feels strange as it heals, particularly if you have the midline incision from sternum to navel. I felt as though I had piano wire between those two points. At other times it feels as if a board's been sown into your chest and belly. And at least a few spots are likely to take weeks and weeks to heal. In my case, it was the union above the sternum, that was asymmetrically closed and left a bigger scar than needed. Also, about ten days post op, when I bent over, something gave a little pop, and I started bleeding at the incision near the navel. It was a small reopening of the suture line, about a quarter of an inch. It sealed shortly after clotting off. Also I was concerned about the symmetry of the closure. The area around the incision was not symmetric, with a dip here, and a rise there. In general the right side somewhat overlapped the left. (Don't let residents or students close you if you can avoid it.) The asymmetry has improved as the weight has come off, and I assume that can all be improved when the scar is revised.

But you'll worry all the time the first six weeks: Do I have a ventral hernia or will I; is it leaking (a seroma or a fistula); is the suture line across the stomach holding, or is it loosening and ulcerating? (I'd think crazy thoughts like, "It must be! I can eat more without discomfort; the suture line must have come apart!" When I asked Sugerman why he didn't transect the stomach the way Dellinger, in Seattle did, he said, "We're confident we can keep the suture line tight." which naturally leaves me wondering if it's come undone.) Maybe it's leaking at one of the other joinures? Am I getting an ulcer at the suture lines? Sometimes your stomach burns, and you think you're getting a gastritis at least.

Then there's enormous gas, and you must be careful at first about what you eat, not to mention the ordeal of a pureed diet for a month.

But it's amazing. Your appetite will change. First it will be markedly diminished. You will be happy with 800 to 1000 calories a day—something you never thought possible. You'll be in ketosis. That will make your breath smell horrible, kind of like moth balls, but the fat in your body cannot be broken down any other way.

Your appetite for sweets will be virtually extinguished. The sight of chocolate won't faze you. You will feel full and satisfied with a little; often too full. And at least once you'll vomit from eating or drinking too quickly.

Best of all, with minimal and reasonable restraint, you will be able to lose weight and keep it off, and it will feel like a miracle compared to your previous attempts to lose weight.

Chapter 10—What It Means

It means freedom

from old demons.

Freedom from hunger.

Freedom from the constant need to restrain yourself.

Freedom from craving and irrational needs.

Freedom from ridicule and the consequent depression and poor self esteem.

Freedom to take pride when you look in the mirror.

Freedom from not being taken seriously because you're a fat slob.

Freedom to buy your clothes off the rack.

Freedom from high blood pressure and the side effects of antihypertensives.

Freedom from high blood sugars, from insulin, and all its paraphernalia, side effects and the increase in hunger it causes.

Freedom from sleep apnea.

Freedom from arthritis.

Freedom to exercise without pain.

Freedom to live a normal life span.

The privilege of seeing your grandchildren.

The privilege of being there to help your children for as long as you possibly can.

It's worth doing.

It's worth getting well.

Godspeed.

0-595-26912-5

www.ingramcontent.com/pod-product-compliance
Lightning Source LLC
Chambersburg PA
CBHW030848180526
45163CB00004B/1497